UP AND RUNNING FOR LIFE

IN NINE EASY STEPS

Bernice Fitzgibbon

Praise for Bernice Fitzgibbon

Up and Running for Life in Nine Easy Steps

Hi Bernice,

I am a 53-year-old, just beginning running, and I just wanted to thank you for your very helpful eBook, *Up and Running for Life*. It was a great read, full of inspiration and very practical things that I would never have thought of, as an inexperienced runner.

I really liked your easy to read style, it was just so friendly, and not daunting at all. There were plenty of technical pointers, you just explained them very well. I also loved your Stretches and Core Strengthening exercises with photos, showing some of the important areas that I need to concentrate on. I intend to implement the Basic Training Program soon, to enable me to achieve my goal of running in a 5 km Fun Run in the not-too-distant future.

Once again Bernice, thanks for a really helpful book.

Kind Regards,
Claire Bathgate
Gosford, NSW

Scan this QR code with your smartphone to visit my website, **UpandRunningforLife.com.**

DISCLAIMER & COPYRIGHT

Your biggest challenge isn't someone else.
It's the ache in your lungs,
the burning in your legs,
and the voice in side you that yells "can't,"
but you don't listen.
You just push harder.
And then you hear the voice whisper "can.
And you discover
that the person you thought you were is
no match for the one you really are.
—Unknown

CONTENTS

ACKNOWLEDGEMENTS

ONE OF THE BEST THINGS I have found in all the years I have been running is the wonderful community spirit amongst runners. It is a big family of like-minded, fun people that extends globally. I have running friends (from all over the world) who I have met just once at an event. But I know if I ever visited their country, I would be made welcome in their homes and vice versa.

Running is a fantastic way to meet people from all walks of life. There is no discrimination, no separateness—we are all runners. It is such an amazing feeling of belonging and being accepted as you are.

Among this amazing group, there are a few people I would like to mention who were great coaches, mentors, and therapists.

First, I have to mention the club I belonged to in Christchurch, New Zealand. Thank you to all the wonderful members, some of whom remain my best friends to this day, even though we are now in different parts of the world.

Pete Watts—club coach and mentor. Although we didn't see eye to eye on many of his decisions he still got me to the line on race day, to prove once again his decision to place me on a particular lap was the right one, if not for me, then for the team.

Don Cameron—another coach and mentor—got me to the finish line on my one and only marathon.

My physiotherapist, Bruce Milne, who fixed me up time and time again after yet another injury. Along with my long suffering general practitioner (GP) and sports doctor, Neil Averis, who also was constantly treating my injuries and getting me back out there to run another day.

I remember one time when I was supposed to be resting my Achilles tendon in my heel, but after several weeks I was so over it. I waited until it was dark and went out for a run. As I run, hobbling along, I hear this voice from a cyclist coming toward me, "That wouldn't be Bernice Fitzgibbon running by any chance?" I couldn't believe I was caught! There was Neil on his bike! Mind you, I was only hurting myself as it took two years and surgery to fix that one.

I think I should add that my injuries were not due to running itself, but me pushing the boundaries, over-training, or ill advice by well-meaning coaches and physios who tried to change my running style to heel strike, which is now considered the wrong way to run.

To all those people a big thank you! This book is in part due to you and your passion for the sport of running. It's a passion I want to share with others who are looking to begin the journey of *Up and Running for Life*.

Have Fun!

Get Fit!

Feel Fabulous!

FOREWORD

I HAVE BEEN LYING in bed with these thoughts going through my head, so I need to get them down.

I love running!

It is my first choice when it comes to exercising, but having said that, I do not run every day. Why? Well, first, life gets in the way, so does the climate. I now live in a climate that is extremely hot and humid early in the day. If you are not a morning person, you will find it difficult to get up at 4:30 am, just to miss the sun and the heat. Second, I am now in my sixties, so I need to train and exercise wisely. I don't want to end up like so many runners who over trained, trained on the wrong surfaces, and didn't eat a proper diet.

I like to cross-train, with at least one day off a week. But this wasn't what I was taught back when I was new to running, well racing, which was the next step on from this book.

I go to the gym two to three times a week, doing mainly classes, such as Body Attack, Body Combat, RPM, Step, Medley, and Pump—not all in the same week. As you will see, there is an imbalance of cardio to stretching, but I do try and stretch after every run and each class. Yoga would be something to seriously think about incorporating into your running, as would weekly or maybe monthly massages.

What you will find in this book is the beginning of my life as a runner, before I even started to compete, but the difference is I now add years of experience to the mix. This is a personal journey, one I am sharing with you in the hopes that you will join me in *UP and Running for Life*

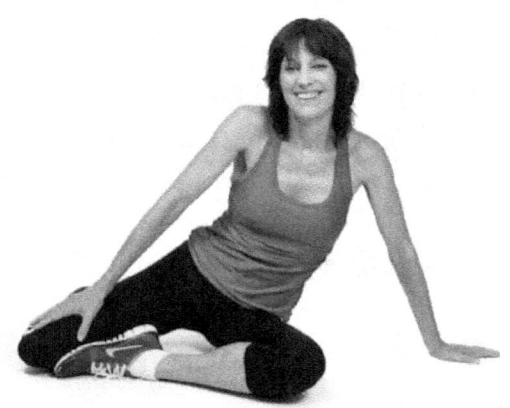

INTRODUCTION

If you run, you are a runner. It doesn't matter how fast or how far. It doesn't matter if today is your first day or if you've been running for twenty years. There is no test to pass, no license to earn, no membership card to get. You just run.

— John Bingham

AS I SAID, I LOVE RUNNING!!! Why do I love running? Because I know it reduces stress, keeps me fit and healthy, and helps me maintain a healthy weight. It also keeps my heart strong and more able to cope with day-to-day living! But most of all, it makes me feel good. It transports me to another dimension where I feel everything is possible, and I am not limited by my external circumstances. There is that heightened awareness of being one with everything—no boundaries, no limitations, just possibilities.

Now, it wasn't like this in the beginning, and, yes, it did take a bit—well a lot—of mental and physical mastery to get me to the above mentioned state of being, but it's so, so worth it.

I first started running at the age of about 10 years, when academically I was at the bottom of the heap. I was labeled dyslexic, which meant little to me, except I was treated differently. I was put in a class one step above children who were intellectually disabled. At that time I needed something to give me some sense of self-worth, as my self-esteem was really low to nonexistent.

It happened by accident, when reluctantly I was entered in a school athletics event by a teacher who could see something in me that I had yet to discover. To my absolute surprise I won every race and most of the field events! This was the beginning of my lifelong passion with running.

I continued running through my high school years and narrowly avoided being expelled several times solely due to my athletic abilities. At 15 years, I ended up being held back a year because of my grades and absences from classes. I decided it was time I left to go out into the big wide world of the working girl.

Move forward ten or so years and three children later. I hadn't run or even exercised since leaving school, but I wanted to lose some of the weight I had gained after having my children. I wanted to do it without needing to diet or, as I had tried, starving myself, then bingeing, another whole story. I also was suffering from what is now called "post-natal depression," along with a high anxiety component. So I was on a rollercoaster ride to nowhere and could see no way out.

A lot of other things went on at this time, but the one thing I remembered from my life was how good I felt when I was running.

So once again I began running, not far at first (as I was so unfit it was an effort to even tie my shoelaces), but I kept going, spurred on by the memory of how great I had felt when I was running. It wasn't that long before the memory was a reality and I was running three to four times a week, slowly at first and short distances, but then faster and farther. What a buzz! I started on my own, then with a friend, until I had a whole group I was running with regularly.

I still remember running my first long-distance run. I was on a high for days. Then I ran my first half-marathon. I loved the way my body reacted to the training—the freedom I felt when I was running on trails through the bush or along the mountainside overlooking the sea. The exhilaration of competing with nature and winning, but most of all the sheer joy I experienced when I ran.

It doesn't matter if you have never run before or you have had a break of some years. It is never too late to start running or begin again.

It doesn't matter if you just want to run to lose weight, get fit, or for the health benefits—now is the right time.

Whatever the reason you want to start running, this book is your formula to success for *UP and Running for Life*.

[1] CHANGE YOUR MIND

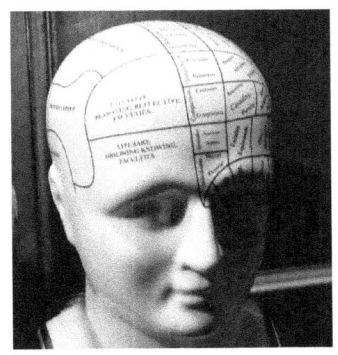

You have powers you never dreamed of. You can do things you never thought you could do. There are no limitations in what you can do except the limitations of your own mind.

—Darwin P. Kingsley

TO START ANYTHING NEW and then continue it for any length of time takes motivation and commitment. Running is no exception. So we need to look at why you have decided to start running.

For me, it was a way to get fit again after having children and also to feel better. I could fit it in with family life without a huge outlay of our limited finances.

I had no set goal in mind, just that it seemed like a good idea at the time. I put on the "Bata Bullets" (a canvas shoe back in my day), a T–shirt (yes, they are still around), and a pair of shorts to head out the door. I had this preconceived idea that I would just pick up where I left off in my early teens!

However, I was now in my mid-twenties, and three children later, the reality was quite different. This, with the fact that the shoes were inadequate along with everything else, about left me feeling disillusioned and terribly sorry for myself.

This was when I needed to reassess my reason for starting to run, as nothing that happened on my first attempt was motivation enough to get me out the door to try again anytime soon.

So what is your motivation to start running?

Is it to get fit? What do you class as getting fit? And what does "getting fit" even mean?! Do you have a measure, that when it is reached, you know you will be fit?

Is it to lose weight? Have you thought about how much weight you want to lose? How soon? Is it measured in weight loss or clothes size or measurements? Is it for a special occasion—your wedding, an anniversary, a class reunion, or another special occasion?

Is it for health reasons? If so, what is your expected health outcome in relation to whatever condition is of concern to you? Is it heart disease, diabetes, obesity, depression, or other illnesses? What measures are you using to say you have achieved what you are after? Is it to feel better, get a good report from your doctor, or to be around for your children or grandchildren?

How strongly do you want this? Have you tried many times and failed? When you start to run, what patterns in your life set you up for success or failure?

Many people fail to address these issues before they start something new, which in turn repeatedly sets them up for failure.

Think about how many times you have started to exercise, and then given up after the first couple of days or weeks. Or think about the number of diets you have been on and have lost the weight to put it (and even more pounds) back on. You don't even get as far as losing the weight! It all becomes too hard.

Why is it that some people succeed in whatever they do and others fail?

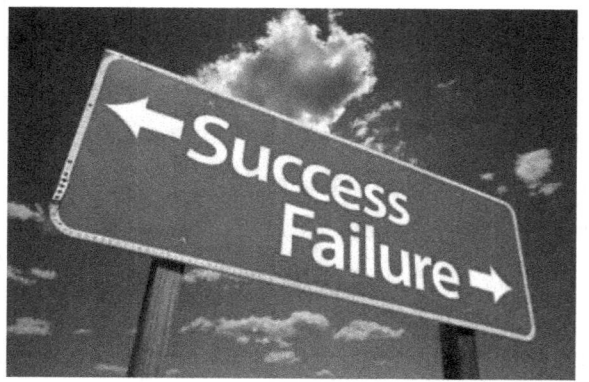

It is all about preconditioning. Something has happened in your early life that has formed a belief that then creates a pattern of behavior, which in turn becomes a habit. The thing is, although the initial belief was established in the conscious mind by something that happened or was said, it is now in the subconscious mind, so you are no longer aware of its existence, yet it is creating your reality over and over again.

Here's the thing, your subconscious mind doesn't like change. It doesn't matter if the behavior you want to change is destructive and doesn't serve you. The sub conscious mind will do everything it can to keep the status quo. So when you first decide, on a conscious level, that you want to start running, or begin some form of exercise, no matter how strong your motivation is, you are going to get some form of internal resistance.

At first, this resistance can be subtle.

"I went out yesterday, so I can have today off."

"It isn't fair to leave the family when I have just arrived home."

You get the picture? Then, if this doesn't work, the resistance becomes less subtle and starts to make even more excuses or blames someone or something to stop you.

If this doesn't work, your subconscious brings out the big guns, so not only does it affect your thoughts and emotions, it also affects you physically! Shortness of breath and a pounding heart are all normal reactions when you are starting a new exercise program. However, all of a sudden these reactions become life-threatening in your mind.

Instead of having the symptoms checked out, your subconscious mind convinces you that they are harming you and you tell yourself:

"Thank goodness, I had the sense to stop this nonsense."

"Why would I want to run? It is way too hard and dangerous. Look, I almost had a heart attack."

Here's the thing, none of this is based on reality; it's only our subconscious minds resisting change. So, how can we get it onboard with what we want to achieve? How do we get it to change its mind, to fit in with what we want to accomplish?

Here's the answer: by being aware of our thoughts. Simple, huh. In theory, yes, but it is essential that we change our habitual thoughts, as this will change our emotions and in turn our patterns of behavior. Listening to our self-chatter—what is running through our conscious minds—will tell us what we believe about ourselves and others. If your self-chatter is that of negativity and self-doubt, you will sabotage yourself without any conscious awareness.

If your underlying belief about yourself is that you are a failure, you can never follow through on anything you started, or you're not good enough to ever be successful at anything, then that is exactly what will show up in your life. All these thoughts are not based in reality but instead are based on a belief you have picked as your own and run with it ever since.

So, anything you try to achieve that doesn't support this core belief will not get past your subconscious filtering system. Only things that support your limiting belief will show up in your life again and again, just to say,

"See, I told you—you are a failure."

The next step is to start to think thoughts that serve the new behavior you want to adopt. The one that says *"You can do anything you set your mind to."* Now I want to add this: do not try to push those negative thoughts out of your mind; acknowledge and give them validation. Say something like this,

"I know you have had my best interest at heart. Thank you for your support, but I would now like your support in my new way of thinking."

By doing this, you are not threatening your subconscious belief, but so you can get past the subconscious filtering system and implant a new core belief! Remember your subconscious mind doesn't like change, so it needs to be distracted and tricked into allowing this new idea in.

About now you are probably saying, "So, what's this got to do with me and beginning to run? I thought you were going to give me the program and I would be away." The problem with that is this: how many diets have people purchased but never followed through on? How many people have tried to quit smoking, but have started smoking again after a short few weeks?

Unless you change your core belief, you will not succeed long term. There is no such thing as willpower. The moment your conscious mind gets distracted, you will automatically go back to the same patterns of behavior you were trying to change. You must change the blueprint in your subconscious mind.

The good news is that once you have done this, it becomes your new pattern of behavior. Anything that reinforces these patterns of behavior will be automatically relayed to the conscious mind and acted on.

In www.changingyourthoughts.com I address these issues. You are no longer controlled by your past and can move forward in the moment. You can change your patterns of behavior to achieve your goals, not just in running, but in every area of your life.

So on to the next step—getting started.

[2] SLOWLY DOES IT!

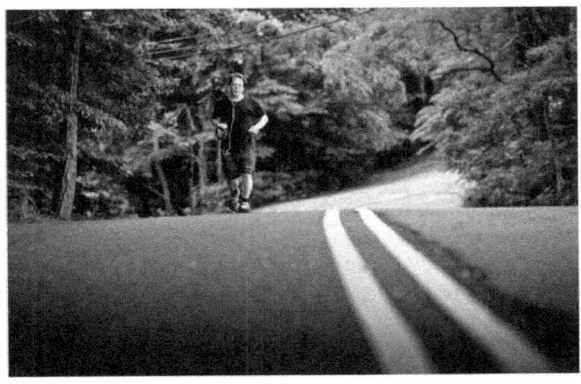

The journey of a thousand miles begins with one step.
—Lao Tzu

RUNNING CAN CHANGE YOUR LIFE and could well be the most important decision you ever make in turning your life around. That being said, it doesn't always seem like fun. Actually, most people start out not enjoying it one little bit.

For one thing, the chances are good that you are out of shape. You're carrying extra weight that you really would like to get rid of but just haven't got around to it. It all seemed too hard and too much effort. Your muscles, if you can find them, are soft and flabby from lack of use. Your joints are stiff and your heart and lungs can't remember what exercise was all about.

Did I say it was going to be easy! No! But if you follow the guidelines, you will wonder why you put it off for so long! You will be looking forward to your next run and the amazing "runner's high" it will bring! But that is down the line a bit!! We must walk before we can run, as the saying goes.

I am asking you to trust me here! The reward is well worth the initial discomfort. Within a brief period of time you will be running consistently for 20 minutes and more.

So, let's get started.

As the chapter title suggests: Slowly Does It! I had run as a child and been good at it, but when I reached my teens I had more important things to do, and I couldn't be bothered with running or doing any exercise. Then I was involved with marriage and children, so by the time I was in my mid-twenties I hadn't done any exercise for a long time.

My first attempt to get back to running was a disaster! I had this memory of what I use to run like when I was a child and thought I was going to just go out and hit the pavement "RUNNING!"

Hit the pavement was right! I would have barely run any distance and the wheels fell off! My lungs were burning, my legs had turned to jelly, and my heart felt like it was jumping out of my chest! I struggled home feeling deflated and hoping no one was watching my disastrous attempt to get back into running.

The next time I went out I was a few days older and wiser and realized I was going to have to start from scratch.

Zero to 5 or 30 Minutes in 12 Weeks

I start by walking quickly for 30 minutes for the first few days. Then I started alternating jogging for a set distance (such as a lamp post, a light pole, a city block, or other designation) with walking for a set distance for 30 minutes. This helped me gain confidence but also begin to condition my mind and body into a new way of being.

Don't think that just because it says "zero to 5" (and I am talking about 30 minutes) that I was going to be able to run all that way in 30 minutes at the end of my 12 weeks. I remember the first time I ran this certain block. I was so excited that the time it took me to run it meant nothing.

However, after that it became a twice-weekly distance and my speed improved until I was extending the runs to 45–60 minutes. But I still hadn't done any hill running or varied the terrain, so this was my next step. Each time I reached my goal, I had another one to aim for. But I didn't go ahead until I had the background conditioning to allow me to move to the next level.

Warming Up, Cooling Down, and Stretching!

To me this is really important, as I am notorious for skipping this and just doing the run. The jury is out on the benefits of stretching. However, it is important to warm up before running. If you are a beginner, walk briskly for 5 minutes before you start to run. If you are a more advanced runner, then start with a light jog for 5 to 10 minutes (or more) depending on the type and length and intensity of training you are going to do.

This is important, as it increases the oxygen supply to the muscles and also warms the muscles for improved flexibility and efficiency. It also slowly raises the heart rate, ensuring minimal stress on your heart. After the run, cool down by walking or jogging for 5–10 minutes to allow your heart rate and breathing to return to normal.

Stretching

There are two types of stretching: static and dynamic.

Static Stretches

Before a run, or for that matter any exercise, you need to get your body prepared. To do this properly you need to get your heart rate up and increase blood flow to the muscles to ensure they are ready for work. Doing a few static stretches is not going to do this and, in fact, can be detrimental to your training and overall performance. Why is this?

According to Jordan D. Metzl, MD, it forces the muscles to relax, which temporarily makes them weaker. This can cause a strength imbalance between opposing muscle groups. For example, stretching your hamstrings can cause them to become significantly weaker than your quads, which in turn might make you more susceptible to injury. They also reduce the blood flow to the muscles and decrease the activity of the central nervous system— that is, it inhibits the brain's ability to communicate with your muscles, which limits your capacity to generate force.

So you should not do static stretches before a run or any exercise requiring muscular strength and force. They are however good for improving overall flexibility, which helps in your day-to-day living.

Again, according to Metzl, stretching twice a day every day is the only way you will gain lasting benefit. He suggests you should do static stretches twice a day, holding the stretch for a minimum of 5 seconds, but 15 to 30 seconds is optimal. There is no need to warm-up the muscles, so for as few as 4 minutes, twice a day, you can improve your flexibility. You only have to stretch the muscle once. You gain no benefit by repeating the stretch.

This brings me to the dynamic stretch.

Dynamic Stretches

What is a dynamic stretch? Dynamic stretching includes active movements of muscle that bring forth a stretch but are not held in the end position. It's when you move a muscle quickly in and out of a stretch, like body-weight lunges.

Your body has many mechanisms that need to be activated and stimulated. When you put your body through a series of stretches while in motion, it sends signals from the brain to the muscle fibers and connective tissues in that area to prepare to do work. Your heart rate and body temperature increase.

Getting good blood flow to the working muscles is critical in order to supply the energy needed to do the work. Along with getting proper blood flow to the muscle fibers and connective tissues, you will also gain more flexibility and increased range of motion. In other words, it improves your active flexibility—the kind required to run. Many studies have shown that dynamic stretching can help increase power, improve flexibility, and increase your range of motion.

According to Metzl if you perform both dynamic and static stretching, some of the flexibility improvements from one stretch will spill over to the other stretch.

So does it help prevent injury? There is no evidence that I could find that suggests that stretching (either static or dynamic) prevents injury. A warm-up before a run or any exercise certainly helps to prepare the body for action, but alone will make little difference in injury prevention. However, combined with other training strategies, it helps in reducing the risk of injury. It's like eating a plate of vegetables and saying you have a healthy diet. Unless you are combining that with other daily healthy food choices, one plate of vegetables does not add up to healthy eating!!

Core Work

It would be remiss of me if I didn't mention core work, as this is an important part of *UP and Running for Life*. This is something I am not good at doing, but I have suffered throughout the years with injuries and time out from running and exercise, which might have been avoided if I had done the core work.

My definition of **core** work is **C**ontinuous, **O**bsessive, **R**epetitive, and **E**ffort. But I have been told I have the wrong attitude to it and should embrace the challenge. Yeah, right! But all joking aside, core work is one of the building blocks to running, or for that matter any exercise program. Core exercises train the muscles in your abdomen, pelvis, lower back, and hips to work in harmony.

Strengthening the core will give you balance and stability, allowing you to efficiently transfer force between the upper and lower body. This ensures that the force you are using to move forward isn't wasted on sideward movement. It ensures optimal body alignment, which in turn adds up to good form and less energy expenditure, which reduces fatigue on longer runs.

Core exercises do not require any equipment and can be done on the floor of any room. It involves not only the abdominal muscles (abs) but other muscles also involved in stabilizing the body.

Running Form

I had no idea about running form when I first started, so I just ran. Now in the beginning this was fine, but as I started increasing my distance I started to have issues, especially with my calves and Achilles tendon. I was a toe runner, meaning my toes strike the ground first, and then my heel, so this was putting a great deal of strain in the above mentioned areas.

I then had a physiotherapist try to retrain me to run as if I had a bucket tied to my buttocks. This meant he wanted me to heel strike first when running, which caused even further injuries and more time out from running.

I am going to discuss form, but again there is the school of thought among runners that as you start to run your body will naturally settle into a running gait. Running is a natural process for the body. It's just we have got out of practice in this modern age.

Here is a guideline for you to follow, if you so wish. It would be remiss of me if I didn't give you a choice:

- **Look ahead of you,** not down at your feet. This keeps you in running form but also is safer, as you can see what is in front of you.

- **Land on your mid-foot.** If you run on your toes, your calves will tighten and become fatigued. If you heel strike, you are over-striding and causing braking. This is a waste of energy and might also cause injury. Try landing on your mid-foot, then roll forward onto your toes.

- **Keep hands at waist level** just brushing gently over the hips at a 90-degree angle. Hands should be relaxed, not with fists clenched. This can be tiring on your arms, shoulders, and neck.

- **Make sure your posture is straight and erect.** Your body is in alignment — shoulders under ears, with your pelvis neutral.

- **Relax your shoulders.** Don't have them hunched up around your ears.

- **Your arms should swing** from the shoulders, not the elbows.

- **Focus on your breathing** — in through the nose and out through the mouth. Breathe from the diaphragm, fully inflating and deflating the lungs.

- **Don't bounce;** try to keep your stride close to the ground with a quick stride turnover. Too much bouncing is a waste of energy and can be hard on your lower body. Think light, as if you are running on a bed of hot coals.

Now this is all wonderful, and you are pumped at the idea of getting started, but "hang on a minute." You might be asking, "When am I going to fit this in?" That's a valid question. I am sure you have heard the saying, "If you want to get something done, ask a busy person." Why? Because they are usually organized, focused, and know how to manage their time effectively. Well, that's what I am told anyway!

When I first started running again, I was getting over what the specialists called "clinical depression with anxiety." I think now it would be called postpartum depression. I had no confidence or self-worth, was not physically fit, carried extra weight, and was emotionally exhausted! I also had three children under the age of five, worked part time at two cleaning jobs, and took in dressmaking to supplement the household income.

I had no idea where or how I would fit the running in, but something inside of me said it was important. The faint memory of how good I felt when I ran spurred me on. So with this faint spark of enthusiasm within me, I began running again.

This was a changing point for me, as it not only benefitted me physically, but also psychologically and spiritually! This was where I gained my physical and emotional strength and confidence to go back to school to get the qualifications I needed to do my nursing education and training.

Later (as a fulltime nursing student, mother, and wife), attending lectures, running children to after-school and weekend activities, keeping house, oh, and hubby happy, plus completing study and assignments, I still fit in running. So how was this possible?

It was possible because I learned how to manage my time effectively. Might I add that time management is not part of my genetic background! In fact, I would have classed myself as one of the best time wasters and procrastinators on the planet.

[3] TIME MANAGEMENT

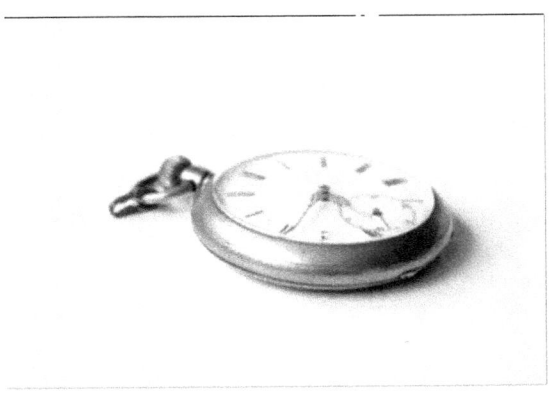

Either you run the day or the day runs you.

—Jim Rohn

FINDING THE TIME TO RUN in an already busy day is always a tricky task, especially when you have a family or a busy work schedule or both. There's that report to finish, a deadline looming, parents evening, or the cake you promised to bake for that weekend, and you haven't been to the supermarket to shop in days. So where to fit a run?

But we are serious about our commitment to start running. YES!! So fit it in, we must. How are we going to do this? As I stated before, it is important to have everyone you can onboard, but even the best-laid plans can go astray. So here is a way of rearranging your life to fit your new running schedule.

You will feel much better if you do run, and as you get better, you will have more energy, sleep better, and any extra weight you are carrying should start to melt away. This is **your** time to switch off from everything else that is going on in your life. It is quite interesting that as you get fitter, you find you are able to cope with more challenges. Things you found stressful before, you seem to handle with much more confidence and a lot less effort. In fact you stop "sweating the small stuff."

So "time management"—not my favorite phrase, but for want of a better one, we will go with this—is something that is necessary if you want to live a less stressful life. This means getting rid of the things that are time wasters. You will know what they are in your life, but examples include

- Spending time on emails that aren't productive or necessary to your day.

- Making phone calls just to have a chat or whine, which is what it ends up being a lot of the time.

- Watch TV mindlessly.

- Not doing your shopping once a week. Then you spend more time going to get things you need for each day.

Get the picture?

There are many time management tools on the Internet, but I want to share some ways you can work your run in without disrupting you routine too much. I want you to succeed, and if making time to run is too difficult, then you might not last the distance. It must become a part of your everyday lifestyle, just like getting up and brushing your teeth is part of your everyday routine.

All it is going to take is 30 minutes, three to four times a week! That's a maximum of two hours a week for your health and wellbeing. Just think about it! This is such a small amount of time when you consider how much time and energy you give to work and to others. The benefits are enormous.

Here are some ideas to get you started:

1. Arrange to run with someone—a relative, friend, or work colleague. You are then accountable, plus if you have an appointment to run, you are more likely to keep it! It is so much easier to run with someone, as the time passes much quicker and it appears to take less effort.

2. Get up an hour earlier, throw your gear on, and head out the door! It might be difficult at first, but it is well worth the effort for the energy you will have during the day. Even if you are not running that day, if you can establish a routine of rising an hour earlier, it will become second nature.

3. Instead of driving your children to school, why not walk them there, and then run home, making sure you are out at least 30 minutes. If it is too far to walk, get to know other parents who might like to run and arrange to have a run from the school after you have dropped the children off. This way you are again accountable but also have running companions.

4. Use your lunch break as running time. It will get you away from your work, and you will have heaps more energy to tackle the afternoon's workload. If you don't have showering facilities at work, your local gym could be an alternative.

5. Pack your running gear the night before, so it is ready in the morning! Then it is one less thing you have to think about.

6. Get dropped off after work at a distance that is 30 minutes from home. Then run home! Or get off the bus a few stops from home to do the same thing.

7. Instead of sitting down to watch TV when you get home, throw your running gear on, and head out for that 30 minute run. You will feel so much better after you have done this. It does take discipline, so if you can arrange to run with someone else, that's all the better! Again, it provides accountability.

8. One of the mothers in our Wednesday running group would arrive with her baby in a pushchair or stroller. If we did hill runs, she would run on the flat and meet up with us, or we would all take turns to "push" up the hill.

9. My daughter, who (surprise, surprise!) runs, has her two children in a stroller and runs them to and from day care. She also works fulltime.

10. It's your turn to babysit. Use this time to get the children out for a bit of fresh air. Have them bike along with you, while you run! Or if they are too young, get a runner's pushchair or stroller. Build stamina and get your run in.

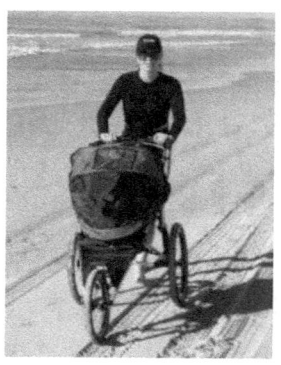

11. Make lunches the night before, if you are planning on making early mornings your time to run. Or use your rest days to prepare meals in advance. Plan your weekly meals and get everyone involved in the preparation.

There are so many other ways you can manage your time so you can fit your run in. Be creative! This is your time.

So far, so good. We have covered mindset and how to recognize and manage the thoughts that sabotage your efforts in the initial stages of this new and wonderful lifestyle change. We have also looked at fitting it in your daily schedule, so it becomes part of your life "habit!" Now it's time to get some commitment. It is time to be accountable.

[4] ACCOUNTABILITY

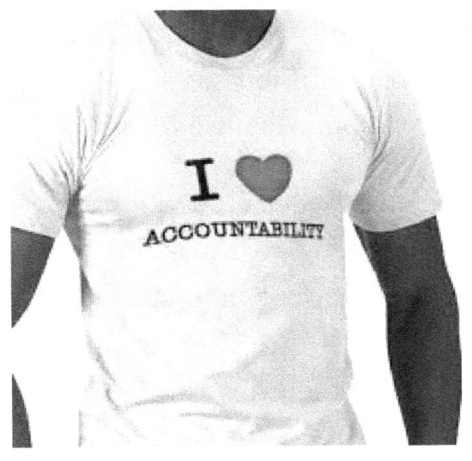

*It is not only what we do, but also what we do not do,
for which we are accountable*

—Molière

DON'T DO IT ALONE! It is so easy to slip back
into old patterns of behavior, especially when you
are first starting out. So what I have to say is an
important part of your training and increases your
likelihood of success in running for life.

Don't do it alone. Unless you are one of those rare people who can decide to do something, then follow through with no help or support, you will need to have someone you are accountable to who is on your team and wants you to succeed.

This is where you need to get your family, friends, work colleagues, and even neighbors onboard! Tell them of your commitment to start running and ask them to support you in your endeavors.

This is important! Because in the early stages, when you are just beginning to run, it is really easy to fall back into old patterns of behavior, especially if your nearest and dearest are not supportive of your running efforts. Sometimes they can be your worst enemy, as they might have a hidden agenda in not wanting you to succeed.

Be aware that you might get some family members or friends who feel threatened. They might think you will change and grow away from them, or you will look and feel better than they do! It is the fear of the unknown: "What if she/he doesn't love me anymore or also expects me to change?". The latter wouldn't be a bad thing. But they don't see it this way.

Even if you do come up against resistance, you need to be strong and find someone who will support you and be on your side. Find a person who is encouraging you and holding you accountable to your program and goals.

The other person you need to be accountable to is yourself. This is where getting your mindset right first is important, and then setting goals that are specific, measureable, and have a time frame. We cover that information in the chapter on "Goal Setting."

You need to have a plan/program designed around your goals and then implement it. It's also essential to reevaluate what is working and what is not, then readjust accordingly!! (This is my nursing background coming out!)

Now, for me (who finds it difficult to stay focused), I need a goal that both expands and excites me. It needs to be something that is challenging, but at the same time I need to believe it is achievable. Please note that I said, "I believe," because if we don't believe we can achieve it, we are already doomed to failure. It goes back to mindset and what we have programmed in our subconscious mind.

Remember you are accountable to yourself and when you try to do something that is outside your comfort zone, or your current level of fitness and experience, you will be more likely to give up at the first hurdle. And there will be hurdles.

Once you have more confidence, you might want to join a running group for further support. There is bound to be one in your local area, or you can even start one yourself. It doesn't matter! What does matter is you have the support you need to keep you going when the going gets tough.

Keeping a diary or journal of your progress is another way to stay accountable. Use one that has dates, so if you miss a run, the entry will be forever blank. On the up side, whenever you follow through, it will be recorded so you have a written record of how far you have come and what you have achieved.

Documenting how you are feeling, both emotionally and physically, helps you become aware of the triggers that influence you to either follow your program or make excuses as to why you didn't do what you intended to do.

There is another good thing about keeping a journal. When you have "down times," you tend to forget how far you've come. You can use your journal to uplift you, not just with your running, but with other areas of your life that you don't feel good about or in control of.

I have had some really dark times in my life when everything appeared bleak. I've looked back in my running journal to get uplifted, and then I realize I am strong and I can succeed.

If you talk about succeeding, any successful person will tell you this: you need to set goals. If you don't have an end in mind, you will never know when you've arrived! So guess what's next! Goal setting.

[5] GOAL SETTING

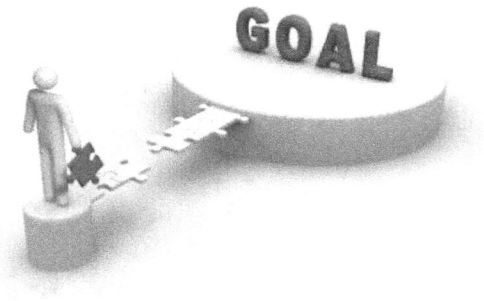

The trouble with not having a goal is that you can spend your life running up and down the field and never score.

—Bill Copeland

FINDING MOTIVATION TO TRAIN on a regular basis and sticking to it isn't always easy! There is, however, a simple formula I found that works, especially when you have a busy schedule and don't feel like making the effort!

This formula (or model) is used in many other areas of life and business—it is the **SMART** formula.

1. Specific

Goals must be specific! If you're not sure what you want to achieve, how are you going to commit time to it? So, what is it you want to achieve!

The other question is why? Why do you want to start to run? That is, what will motivate you to keep going through the tough times in your training?

So your goal might look like this:

To run continually for 30 minutes in six weeks.

2. Measurable

Goals need to be measurable. You need to be able to measure your progress, so you know you are improving and are going to meet your expected outcome within the timeframe.

3. Attractive

This is different from the usual "A" of the SMART formula (which is the word "Appropriate"). I learned this alternative word from an Inspired Spirit Coaching Academy course while training to be a transformational coach. If something isn't attractive to you and doesn't inspire you, then you are more likely to give up at the first hurdle. So, in planning your goal, make sure it has elements that are motivating and inspiring to you.

4. Realistic

It must be something you can achieve with the resources and the time restraints you have now. You also have to believe you can achieve this goal, so if it isn't something that in your mind is realistic, then you will not achieve it.

5. Timely

Goals need to have a timeframe. Without this, how are you going to achieve an expected outcome? Hey, you could say "I will run continuously for 20 minutes one day." What motivation is that, and where is the accountability we talked about earlier?

Once you have your goal, it is time to move to the action side of the goal setting, which includes planning, implementation, and reevaluating.

6. Planning

How are you going to meet your goals? This is where the program comes into it. It needs to have simple, easy-to-follow, and commit-to steps in order to achieve your goals. So that could be four to six weeks of increased effort and distance.

7. Implementation!

Now all of the above ideas are useless if they are not implemented. You need to take action. It is consistent action, however small, that is going to get you to your desired outcome. That is why the "WHY!" is important. If you don't know why you want to start running, then you are setting yourself up for failure and that is not what you want.

8. Re-evaluate

The final step is to re-evaluate your progress. Ask yourself:

- Has my goal been unrealistic to my level of fitness or my other commitments?
- Have I set myself up for failure?

- How can I change it around so it works for me?

Flexibility is important, as things do come up in life. You have deadlines to meet, your family needs something, or you suffer an injury or illness.

On the other hand, you might have met your goal much earlier than your original timeframe. This is when you can move the goalpost and extend yourself further.

This brings me to the next important component to any goal; you need to be setting new ones. Move the goalpost. That is why having short-term goals and long-term goals are important. When you reach one milestone, you need to have your next one in place, so you keep moving forward.

Having a weekly, monthly, and yearly planner (with all the different types of training you can do, the distances and upcoming events/races you are aiming for) is an excellent motivator and way of keeping track of your progress. You will be able to plan for a specific race in your area, be it your first race, a half-marathon, or a marathon. Nothing is more motivating than that.

My first race was the Christchurch half-marathon. I had been running for more than a year, building for this race. I started with the 5-kilometer (km) circuit around the outskirts of my hometown. It took me three months of training for three times a week, extending my distance each week by 10 minutes.

Then I started finding other runs that were longer, trying to run off the road and as often as possible on tracks, grass verge, or beach. I did start running with a friend for a while, but she was working different shifts and quite often couldn't make it. At this time most of my running was on the flat to slightly undulating. I hadn't had the courage to try the hills, too scary.

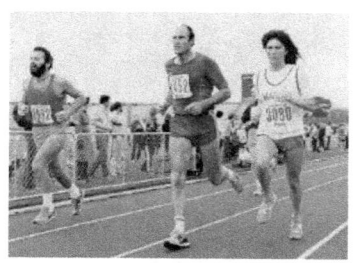

At about five to six months, I was running 10–12 km and feeling good, with so much more energy, despite the fact I was studying, running a house, and managing my family. My confidence had soared, which reflected in all areas of my life. By the time I ran the half-marathon, I still had not run a half-marathon distance in training. Despite this, I still completed the distance with a certificate and photo to prove it.

So what is next? How can we make this more interesting, thereby increasing the chances of success!! Simple, mixing it up!

[6] MIXING IT UP!

Running gives freedom, when you run you can determine your own tempo, you can choose your own course and think whatever you want, nobody tells you what to do.

—Nina Kuscik

VARIETY IS THE SPICE of life, but it is also a way of varying your running, using different muscles in your body and developing overall cardiovascular fitness, muscle tone, strength, and flexibility. There are also the psychological benefits of mixing it up.

When you first start out, don't complicate it. Just follow the basic beginner plan. But as you get fitter, more confident, and can see some positive changes, then you will want to start mixing it up

So let's start with the venue, or where you are going to run. At first you will probably run close to home or somewhere that is easy to get to but maybe away from the neighbors. This depends on how self-conscious you are about being seen, but also if you have teamed up with others on the same journey to *UP and Running for Life* and are meeting them somewhere for a run.

Once you have a little more confidence, then you can start to explore your area. Some places to run could include these areas:

- local parks
- beaches
- waterfront walkways
- forest tracks
- hills and mountain roads
- tracks

All these various terrains use different muscle groups, so you are not developing some leg muscles and leaving other leg muscles weak. It is also helping with strength and stability.

Running on hills is good for cardiovascular fitness, strength, and resistance training on the uphill, and stretching and lengthening your stride plus speed (if you want too) on the downhill. You need to be careful running downhill, as it is extremely hard on your muscular-skeletal system. I loved the downhill lap in races, but it took me longer to recover than any of the other runners on the team.

Pace is the next thing in the mix. When you begin, a walk-a-bit, run-a-bit mix is about all you will be up to, and this is all good. We don't want you to fall apart or feel disillusioned because you only ran a short distance and then collapsed, gasping for air. My trick!!! Even if you can only walk at a brisk pace initially for 20 minutes, that is still good. You will soon improve. Don't try to rush it. It is better to stay on a lower level for several more weeks than force yourself to go farther and faster. This is when injuries happen.

Once you are running consistently for 20 minutes or more, then increasing the distance and time on your feet is the next step. At this stage in your running, you are building background stamina and strength that you are going to need. This is your base training or aerobic conditioning before you start to introduce other forms of training. There is no substitute for time on your feet. This is the foundation of all running programs.

Once you have the base and are able to run three to four days a week for up to an hour or more, you can start to introduce some effort or tempo runs. For me, remembering this is not a technical book, there are three different methods I use:

1. Interval or fartlek training. This is a form of running in which there are high intensity bursts followed by slow recovery phases throughout the duration of a run. In my day we called it fartlek, Swedish for "speed play." This can be as casual or as intense as you want it to be. Remember, the run/walk routine or run for 20 seconds, walk for 20 seconds? Well, you can do this same routine, but pick up the intensity, as it is up to you. The idea of interval training is to improve performance, speed, and endurance. (It also adds interest and variety.)

2. Speed work or repetitions. This is running at speed and doing a certain number of repetitions (reps) with a short rest between! The farther the distance you are planning on racing, the longer the reps should be. This will really start to wake up those fast-twitch muscles.

3. Pace or tempo running/ time trials. This is to learn to run consistently at a certain pace over a certain distance. It also gives you a gauge to go by when training for a certain race, so you can see how you are doing over time. If you are not improving, or are going backward, you will need to reexamine your training program and adjust it accordingly.

There is a whole new language of running, and it is something I am not going to discuss in this book. However, you will find a list of resources at the end, and I will cover this in the next book of the UP and Running for Life series, but this is just to get you started!

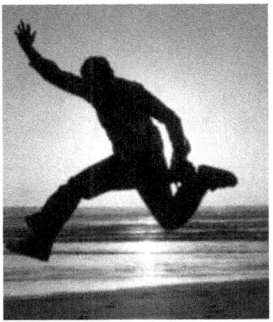

I know you are just starting out and might be thinking "I can't even run yet, let alone do all this type of training." But you will be surprised how quickly you will be running consistently for 30 minutes and be looking for new challenges. Always keep in mind, though, that the background or base work is the foundation for all other forms of running. Don't try to rush ahead too quickly or you will end up injured.

Finally, should you train indoors on a treadmill or in the great outdoors? For me, there is no competition, I love running outdoors, but it isn't for everyone. So if you are one of those people who would prefer to get started in the privacy of their own home and buy treadmill, that's great. Or you can join a local gym and use the equipment, the principles are the same.

If you want the treadmill to be as close as it would be running outdoors and you also want to burn the same number of calories for the time and effort, you will need to have the incline set to about a 1 percent gradient. If your intention is to get fit enough to run your first fun run, I would have said that you really need to have done some outdoor running. However, I met a women who has run marathons on all seven continents (including Antarctica) and because of her work location, she does most of her training on a treadmill.

Anyway, the choice is yours, but if you do decide the treadmill is the way to go, make sure you have a good selection of music to listen to, as it can be quite boring and I don't want you to give up.

Next, let's discuss what to wear. What will you need to get started on this new way of life?

[7] CLOTHES AND EQUIPMENT

You always have a choice, you can throw in the towel or you can use it to wipe the sweat of your face.

—Unknown

WELL, HERE WE ARE the big fashion statement corner of *UP and Running for Life*.

If you are a beginning runner, here's what you need:

- A pair of well-fitting shoes to suit you
- A supportive sports bra or crop top (women)
- A pair of comfortable shorts or tights
- A T-shirt or top of your choice

Not what you expected? We are here to get you "running for life" and if it is going to be too difficult, too expensive, or too "How do I look?" you might never get to first base. KISS is the principle—"Keep It Simply Simple!"

It will depend where you live and at what time of year you start your UP and Running for Life steps, so this will need addressing. However, to begin, we are trying to make it easy for you.

Shoes

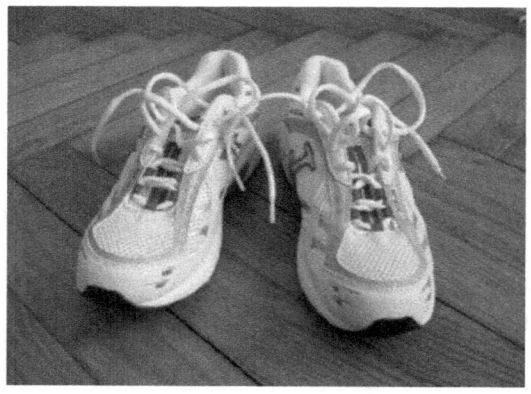

I can't express enough the importance of having good shoes! Gone are the days when I first started running, when the good old Bata Bullet was the shoe of choice. Mind, minimalistic running is all in vogue now, but whatever you choose you need to see the experts.

We have sophistication now. You need to get the right running shoe for you. Not just your foot, but also for how you run. Yes, run! Because that is what you are doing all this for. I have been through many a shoe in my running lifetime to know, if it doesn't suit my running style, I have issues.

I have had physios trying to correct my running style so I could have the "perfect" gait, which they thought was that I should land on my heels first, then roll gracefully to my toes into the next perfect stride. This led to one injury after another, as my body was not designed to run this way. Nor is anyone else's body, for that matter.

Anyway, enough of me! Let's focus on the right shoe for you. I don't know how you run, so I will refer you to the experts who fit shoes for a living. There are specialist shoe stores in your area that can check your running or walking style, and this is where you should start.

There are many top brands of shoes that specialize in every type of foot, so check them out. As you get more into running, the same shoe you start with might not suit you later in your running life.

I am not going to get into all the ins and outs of running shoes, as there are so many different brands and styles available to suit any running style or preference. There are shoes that give full support and stability to ones that are designed as if you were running barefoot. I have tried just about every type of shoe and have settled for a neutral last, light but stable, fit for training and trail running, but a lightweight minimal shoe for road racing and spikes for cross-country racing.

Socks are also something to choose carefully, as some can actually cause blisters. Again, there are so many brands of sports socks, pick one that is comfortable for you.

Sports Bra

For women, a good fitting sports bra or crop top is essential, so go to a store that specializes in sportswear. You need a bra to fit you properly to give maximum support and feel comfortable. When I first started, I wore a Bendon bra from the orchid collection. If I remember, it was pink and although it looked pretty, it wasn't comfortable for running and certainly didn't give me the support I needed.

I actually did my first cross-country relay race in it. I had pinned the number on the wrong side of my singlet, so at the start line, I had to whip it off in front of everyone, turn it around so it was now on back to front, just as the runner came in to tag me and I was on my way. Everyone there remembered the incident and the bra, but nothing about my run.

Now back to business. Other than that, there is so much to choose from, but as a beginner, as long as it is comfortable and serves the purpose you need it for, then anything goes. We want you running now, not after weeks of shopping for the just right running fashion accessory.

Other Needs

Let's discuss protection from the sun. Yes, I know you absolutely need your vitamin D, but let's do it in a controlled manner.

You can choose head gear, maybe a cap of some kind and be sure to use sunblock. If you are running in the cooler part of the day, which is recommended, sunscreen might not be necessary. But at any other time, it is important to protect your skin.

If you are running in the colder part of the year or in a climate that is relatively cold, then you will need to wear the appropriate clothing for your conditions.

Eye protection is also important as the sun's rays can damage the eyes, and that is the last thing you want. Choose a good pair of sunglasses that is comfortable and suitable for running. Close-fitting, wraparound shades are best, as they don't block your vision. Check out different sports brands of sunglasses until you find a pair that fits your face and is comfortable to wear. Transitional lenses are great, as you can be running in the shade or full sunlight, and they will adjust accordingly.

Not essential to have, but useful, is a watch. A simple one will do, but if you want to know how many calories you have burned or the distance you covered, then you might purchase a watch with these different functionalities. There are gadgets to suit everyone, but none of them is essential to begin with.

You can also download an app on your phone that will beat out your stride or pace so you get your cadence right. It's not half as good as music, and I believe now-a-days you can download music that is designed for running at pace. It would seem to me to be a better way of motivating you to run. It's also a great way to distract your mind and the self-chatter that tells you that this is too hard.

I use to run with a Walkman in a specially designed belt and big thick headphones to the sounds of '80s music. Things have certainly changed.

Anyway moving along—the next area to address is what powers your engine and keeps it operating to maximum performance: nutrition and hydration.

[8] Nutrition and Hydration

The power of the human will to compete and the drive to excel beyond the body's normal capabilities is most beautifully demonstrated in the arena of sport.

—Aimee Mullins

THIS IS THE ONE STEP I find the hardest to address, as I have been running for many years and still don't have the right nutritional plan to suit everyone. However, there is one fundamental thing that every good nutritional plan should have and that is balance.

Now I am not talking about a rigid eating plan here, but it is important to get the necessary nutrients for a healthy body.

There is so much information out there on what you should or shouldn't eat, how often, how much, and if you should take supplements. All have valid scientific evidence supporting their claims, but when it comes down to it, everyone is different and what might suit one person might not suit another.

I remember many years ago when I was first dating my partner, Robert. I was his support crew on a six-day race. Now this was no ordinary race that went from point A to point B, no! It was around and around a 400 meter track for six days. The runner went four hours one way, and then a bell would ring and everyone would turn and run in the other direction. The idea was the runner who covered the most distance in the time was the winner.

Anyway, as I said, I was his one and only support crew member and was responsible for everything from cooking, keeping records, getting supplies, and tending to all his aches and pains—nursing duties. I had to keep an accurate record of his daily food intake following a strict diet that had been set by long-distant runners and research papers written on the subject of nutrition for distance running. This involved me preparing carbohydrate-loaded meals at regular intervals among all my other tasks.

Despite following the menu to the letter, Robert was feeling weak and extremely tired, finding he had to stop frequently, something he couldn't afford to do. So by the third day he was considering calling it quits!

It was at this time (4:00 am to be exact) that the cooker I was preparing his porridge on gave up. I sat there crying, looking at the watery mess in the pot and wondering what I was going to do. After giving Robert his watery porridge, I crashed. The following morning I went to the caravan that was supplying food for the support people and bought a large steak sandwich with all the extras and gave it to him.

He was reluctant to eat it, as this food didn't follow all the findings of the research. I advised him that if he wanted the relationship to go any further, he would eat it! He saw my point of view and did so. Well surprise, surprise!!! His energy levels rose and he felt better than he had for days.

So from then on it was steak sandwiches, bacon and eggs, and everything in between, as long as I didn't have to cook it! He didn't win, but stayed the distance, something that might not have happened if he had continued to stick to his original diet!

So this is what I mean when I say that there is no one rule that fits every person, you need to listen to what your body tells you and adjust your diet to suit. Making smart choices about the type, time, and quantity of food you eat is important to everyone's well-being, but even more so, once you start to exercise.

Your body requires energy (calories/kilojoules) to function, and it gets this from the food you eat! If you are getting your daily requirements, your weight should remain stable and you should have the energy to comfortably do all the activities of your daily living.

If, however, you are either not getting enough or too much of a good thing, over time this will start to show in weight gain or difficulty managing your day-to-day activities as in Roberts case.

What constitutes a balanced diet, which has the flexibility to change as your requirements change?

Let's look at what a balanced diet contains by looking at the constituents or components:

- energy, for example, calories /kilojoules
- proteins

- fat
- carbohydrates
- vitamins and minerals
- fiber
-

Let's briefly look at each one of these components.

Energy

Your body's primary need, apart from water, is energy. This is signaled by the body as hunger. The amount of energy required is measured in calories or kilojoules, depending on your measuring system! A thousand calories = 1 kilocalorie (kcal), which is what most people are referring to when they are counting calories.

The other measure is in joules:

1,000 joules = 1 kilojoule (kj), therefore 1 kcal=4.2 kj

We need energy for life, including all the voluntary activities, such as movement and things we can observe. We also need energy for involuntary functions that go on inside the body that we can't see but are essential to growth, such as body maintenance and repair, temperature regulation, breathing, digestion and absorption, and much more.

The rate at which you use this energy is known as your metabolic rate. Your energy requirements change at different stages in your life. For example, growth requires much more energy, as does physical exertion, so when you exercise or do any kind of physical activity requiring effort, your energy requirements are going to increase! Now, women, I hate to tell you, but not everyone is made equal— men require more energy per body weight than women!! Not fair, but this is because men have more fat-free mass (FFM) than their female counterparts.

The FFM determines how many calories you burn, Fat burns few calories, therefore men require more calories per day than a woman of the same age and weight!!

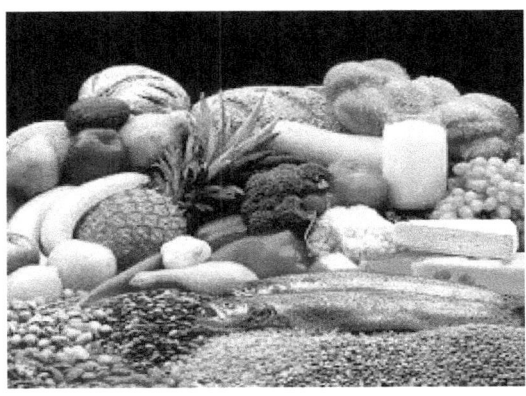

What a daily balanced diet should contain are the following items:

1. fruits and vegetables
2. bread, cereal, pasta, potatoes (carbohydrates)
3. meat, fish and alternatives, for example, tofu (protein food)
4. milk and dairy products
5. food containing unsaturated fats, for example, nuts, avocados.

If you eat a balanced diet, you should get all the vitamins, minerals, and nutrients to meet your body's daily needs. Buying organic can increase your chances of the supply being unpolluted. Also eating fresh food, rather than refined and processed food, will give you a better chance of meeting your body requirements.

So here are the components required by our bodies to meet the activities of daily living. You have two types of nutrients. Your macro nutrients and your micro nutrients.

Macro Nutrients

Proteins

Proteins are the building blocks of your body. Without them, you wouldn't be able to replace and repair body cells.

Protein is a major component of structural tissues, such as skin and collagen, which is found in connective tissue, such as tendons and ligaments. Blood requires protein as does your immune system. All enzymes are proteins. Proteins are made up of amino acids. There are three types, essential, nonessential, and conditional amino acids. Essential amino acids cannot be made by the body, so they must be obtained from the food we eat. It is recommended that approximately 25–30 percent of energy comes from proteins.

Sources of protein are meat, fish, and alternatives, such as tofu.

Carbohydrates, Sugars, Starches, Fiber

Carbohydrates (carbs) are the body's main source of fuel. This means 50–65 percent of our daily requirements need to come from carbs in maintaining our daily energy needs.

When extra demand is placed on the body, as happens during times of physical or emotional stress, the amount required is at the upper end of 65 percent or more. When carbohydrates are broken down to their simplest form, they can be used by the cells in the body as fuel. Your brain is almost entirely dependent on it for all functions, including thinking. One gram of carbohydrate equals 17 kj or 4 cal.

It depends on the type of carbs you eat to determine how much time it will take to break the food down to useable energy or fuel for the body. High glycemic index (GI) foods, such as fruit, biscuits, and sports drinks, will break down and be absorbed into the blood stream for utilization much faster than low GI foods, such as multigrain breads, rice, and pasta.

High GI foods might be beneficial at times when your energy needs are greater, for example, one to two hours pre- and post-training sessions or races. Low GI foods might be more beneficial to have four to five hours pre- and post-exercise.

Excess sugars are stored in the skeletal muscles and liver as glycogen. These stores are mobilized if you are not getting enough energy from your diet or if you require energy quickly, such as when you are exercising. If the stores are full, sugar is converted to fat and stored as adipose tissue around the body. If carbohydrate stores are inadequate to meet your daily needs, this can result in fatigue, reduced training ability or performance, and impaired immune system function, which can lead to illness, such as colds and flus.

Fats

Fats are a necessary part of your diet for four reasons:

1. They make your food taste better.
2. They are a concentrated source of energy.
3. They provide fat-soluble vitamins and essential fatty acids.
4. They provide insulation, protection, cushioning, and cell protection

There are two types of fats: saturated and unsaturated fats. Saturated fats are those derived from animals; unsaturated fats are derived from vegetables. Usually saturated fats are more solid at room temperature than unsaturated fats. There are some exceptions to the rule, such as coconut oil, which is a saturated fat and a liquid.

Saturated Fats

Also known as "bad fats," this category also includes "trans fats." These fats are the ones that cause health issues, such as obesity, coronary heart disease, type II diabetes, hypertension, and stroke, to name a few. These fats are derived from animals and are usually solid at room temperature. They contain LDL or VLDL cholesterol, which clogs the arteries.

Essential Fatty Acids

Most fatty acids are made in the body, but there are two that must be supplied for the body to work properly. They are also important in transporting and breaking down cholesterol and are used in the manufacture of other chemicals in the body and, of course, fat-soluble vitamins.

Micro Nutrients

Vitamins and Minerals

One would hope that if you eat a balanced diet you get all the vitamins and minerals to meet your body's daily requirements. But with modern diets, food processing, pollution, and other impacts, this isn't always the case. So you might need to take supplements.

There is much information about what the recommended daily intake should be. If you buy supplements from a reputable supplier, a counselor will be able to advise you about the brands and which vitamins and minerals will best suit your specific needs.

Hydration

Your body needs to be well-hydrated in order to function. Our bodies are 75 percent water, so just a loss of 2 percent (through metabolic activity during exercise) will have a negative effect on performance and health.

The effects of dehydration during exercise are related to the amount of fluid loss. In warmer climates this loss is going to be much greater than in cool climates or in the cooler months! The amount of effort is also going to affect the amount of fluid loss during your run.

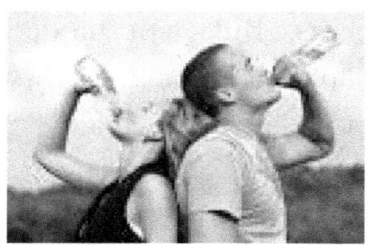

Carrying water with you, or knowing where you can get a drink on your run, is important, but so is being well-hydrated before your run. Problems are more likely to arise during a run if you are already dehydrated before you begin.

Be sure to rehydrate following your run, as this will help your body flush out the chemicals released during exercise. It will also carry nutrients via the circulatory system to the muscles and remove waste, a byproduct of exercising. If you are feeling thirsty, chances are you are already dehydrated.

The five common causes of dehydration are:

1. inadequate fluid intake; something I'm guilty of!

2. failure to replace fluid loss during and after exercising

3. excess sweating

4. exercising in dry, hot weather

5. drinking only when you feel thirsty

Because we all sweat at different rates, for many reasons, it is difficult to give a specific recommendation on the amount and type of hydration required. Anything from 2 to 3 liters or gallons a day might be needed, especially in warmer climates. But if you sweat a lot, you are going to need to replace that fluid!

I ran with a guy who used the "pee test" to monitor his level of hydration! He would drink until his urine was almost clear and maintain this throughout the day! If he wasn't going to the toilet as often as he usually did and the urine color was darker, he would drink more fluids! That is if he hadn't just taken a multivitamin!

The only other issue I will touch on here is sports drinks. There are many effective sports drinks on the market these days, and most of them are good. The reason you would be drinking a sports drink is to replenish your body's energy levels and replace essential minerals that you have lost during exercise. When you are starting out, you really won't need these types of drinks. Remember, they carry a high calorie value that if you are running to lose weight you really don't need.

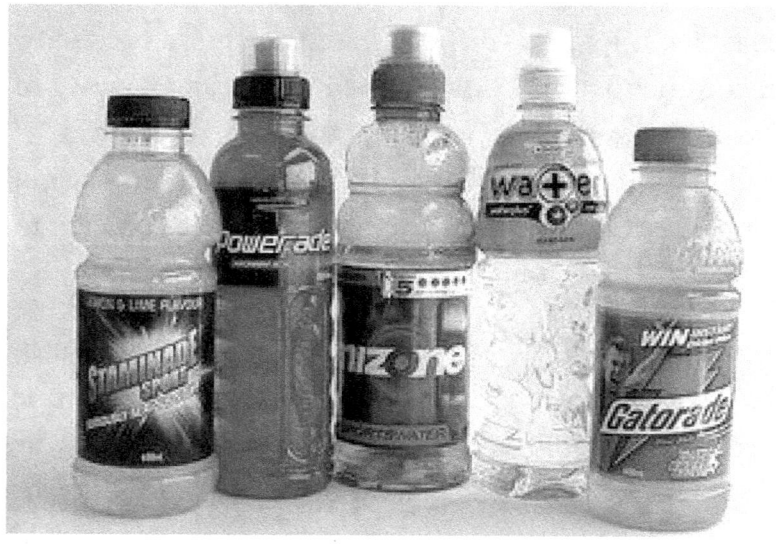

There are three types of sports drinks.

1. **Isotonic**—the same concentration as normal body fluid, so it's absorbed easily; they would typically contain 4–8 grams of carbohydrates per 100 milliliters.

2. **Hypotonic**—less concentrated than normal body fluid, so it is quickly absorbed by the body; these would typically contain fewer than 4 grams per 100 milliliters.

3. **Hypertonic**—more concentrated than the normal body fluid, so it is absorbed more slowly; these would have a concentration greater than 8 grams of carbohydrates per 100 milliliters.

There are many sites on the Internet to access more information on this subject, so check them out. There are lists at the back of this book, if you want to know more. However, it's beyond the scope of this book, keeping in mind that this is not a technical book.

[9] REST AND SLEEP

Courage doesn't always roar, sometimes courage is a quiet voice at the end of the day saying I will try again tomorrow.

—Mary Ann Radmacher

WHY IS REST AND SLEEP an important part of the nine easy steps to *UP and Running for Life*? Aren't we supposed to be getting fit here? So what does rest and sleep have to do with that.

The simple answer is that rest days are critical to running performance, whether you are just a beginner or an elite runner.

Rest is physically necessary so that the muscles can repair, rebuild, and strengthen. Built-in rest days help maintain a better balance between home life and work life, and your fitness goals and balance is what this is all about!

So what happens during rest and recovery?

The body adapts to the stress of exercise and the real training effects taking place. It also allows the body time to replenish energy stores and repair damaged tissues. Believe me, when you are first starting out you will find muscles you never thought you had in places you didn't know existed, so initially they are going to need time to adapt to this new experience.

Any exercise causes changes in the body, such as muscle tissue breakdown and the depletion of energy stores (muscle glycogen) and fluid loss. Rest allows these stores to be replenished and tissue repair to occur. Without sufficient time to repair and replenish, the body will continue to breakdown, and this then puts you at risk of injury. It also can compromise your immune system, increasing your vulnerability to illness.

Although you are just starting out or just getting back into running after a long break, the principles are the same as a person who has been running for some time.

As this is nine easy steps to *UP and Running for Life*, we want you to stay the distance, so although you can't see the day when you could be tempted to over train, as you get fitter, this can easily happen. Even as a beginner you need to plan ahead and have all the tools available to give you the best chance of success.

When you first start to run ,you will still need to have a warm-up and cool-down period. This gets your body ready for the run and then helps it recover from the run. The latter allows the soft tissues (muscles, tendons, and ligaments) time to repair and remove chemicals that have built up as a result of cell activity during the run.

Adaption to exercise is when we undergo the stress of physical exercise and our bodies adapt and become more efficient. It is like learning a new skill. At first it is difficult, but over time it becomes second nature. Remember the "over time" bit and don't expect to feel good after your first few runs. We don't want you quitting before you start to see the benefits you will gain by persevering.

There are limits as to how much stress the body can tolerate before it breaks down and risks injury. Doing too much, too quickly will result in injury or muscle damage, but doing too little, too slowly will not result in any improvement. This is why we have set up specific training programs that increase time and intensity at a planned rate, allowing for rest days throughout the program.

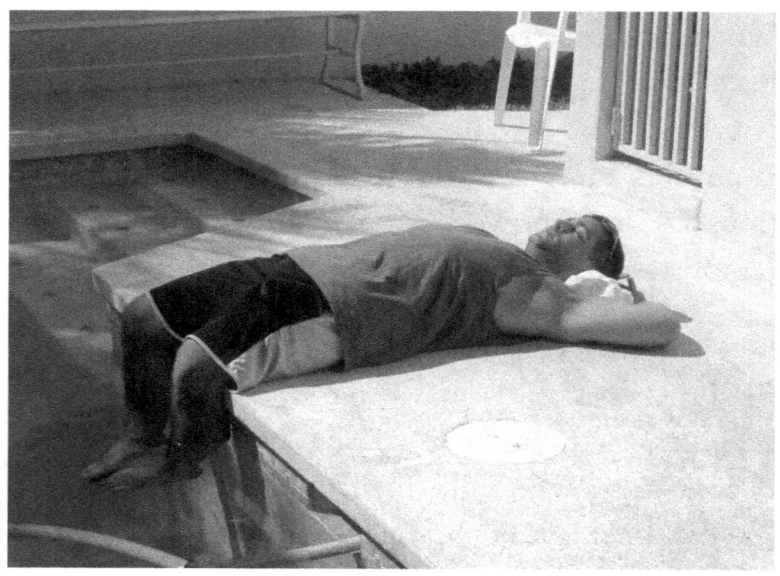

Sleep is the other area that can hinder your progress and overall wellbeing. In most cases, one to two nights of sleep deprivation shouldn't impact your training, but if you are consistently getting inadequate sleep it can result in changes to your hormone levels, especially those relating to stress, muscle recovery, and mood.

Although little is known about the complexities of sleep, some research indicates that sleep deprivation can lead to increased cortisol levels, a stress hormone, with a decrease in the human growth hormone, which is active during tissue repair and decreased glycogen synthesis.

Suffice it to say that rest and sleep play a major role in your ability to be a runner for life.

[10] ADAPTATION

If we all did the things we are capable of doing we would literally astound ourselves.

—Thomas Edison

NOW SOMETHING I HAVE BRIEFLY touched on in a roundabout way, but not really explained, is the body's ability to adapt to its environment. I hear so many people say, "I can't do that," and then proceed to tell the story to justify the reason why they can't do something. To them it is the truth, it is what they believe, but I am here to challenge that belief, to get you to question what you have accepted as your truth.

As this book about running, I am looking at it from the context of this statement, "I can't run, because . . . " and really look at where that comes from. And, yes, there will be some science to help you rethink what you believe.

Think about the 4-minute mile. Up until 1954 no one had ever run a mile in less than 4 minutes. Then on May 6, 1954, a British runner, by the name of Roger Bannister, did just that. Up until then it was believed the human body was not capable of running at such speed.

It wasn't long after that, that the 4-minute mile was being broken consistently. It just took that shift in consciousness and someone to defy the odds and then others followed. Now most fairly good runners can run a mile in less than 4 minutes.

The body has an amazing ability to adapt to what is placed on it. This couldn't be more so when it comes to exercise and running.

Adaptation refers to the body's physiological response to training. As we increase the load on the body, the body reacts by increasing its ability to cope with that load. When you are new to running, you will find that you progress fairly quickly. That is, if you are reasonably healthy and don't have any underlying issues that might require medical intervention, in which case you will need to get medical clearance to start any new exercise program. I am making an assumption that you are able to start running, so as a beginner your progression from jogging for 30 seconds in the walk/run phase will soon progress to running 30 minutes without a break.

During this time, there will be physiological changes happening in different systems in your body. The cardiovascular and respiratory systems increase output and volume capacity, and the number of capillaries supplying the muscles increases. As the demand for oxygen and nutrients to the body increases, so does the efficiency of the cardiovascular and respiratory systems.

The muscular-skeletal system adapts to cope with the force and weight-bearing load placed on it. The muscles develop in strength initially and increase in size over time. This is required as the muscles generate the force for propulsion and absorb the impact when running. The bones and joints also need to adapt to the load. When sufficient stress is placed on a bone, new bone is deposited to the area, thus giving the bone more strength.

The nervous system gives the signals to the muscles to contract. No signal, no contraction. It is the intensity, duration, and timing that determines how long and how hard the muscle will contract.

There are many other processes going on with the body that contributes to its ability to change and adapt to its environment. Some happen fairly quickly, while others take millions of years.

The thing is that our bodies adapt over time. If you are a beginning runner, you will experience fairly rapid change in the first few weeks, but as your body adapts, you will need to challenge yourself further.

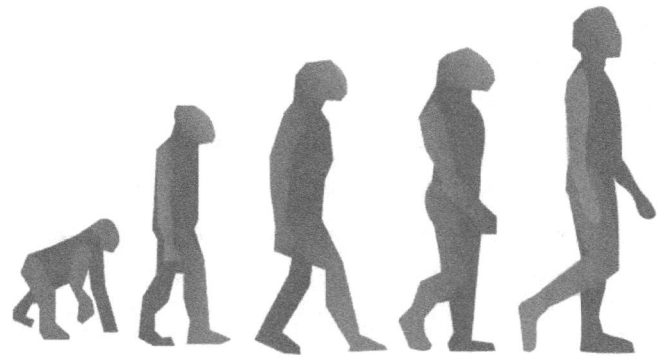

[11] Getting Started Beginner's Program!

This program isn't the only one out there by any stretch, but it is close to the one I used when I was first getting started. Now I had run before, so my body did have some memory of what it was like and what to expect, even if it didn't like it or respond the way I would have liked, at first.

During the early stages, when you are in the walk/run phase, easy does it, just jog at a pace that feels comfortable for you. You will soon start increasing your running time and then your pace will also naturally increase.

Always do a warm up and cool down, for example, walk 5 minutes and then you might want to do some light stretches, but this is optional as there is no scientific evidence that stretching before your run prevents injury or is of any value to your overall performance. Now begin the program followed by a 5-minute cool down and some light stretches.

PHASE ONE: Minimum of Four Weeks

Walk and jog 15–20 minutes per day, four days a week. For example, Monday, Wednesday, Friday, and one day on the weekend.

PHASE TWO: Minimum of Four Weeks

Jog for 15–20 minutes per day, four days a week.

PHASE THREE: Minimum of Four Weeks

Jog 15–20 minutes on two days, say Monday and Friday; and then 30 minutes on two days, say Wednesday and one weekend day.

You should now be able to run 30 minutes without stopping. Congratulations!

Now you will be ready to increase your distance and time on your feet, or you might wish to stay at level three for a bit longer; it is entirely up to you.

PHASE FOUR: Minimum of Four Weeks

Jog on four to five days a week, as follows:

Monday-Tuesday-Thursday-Saturday-Sunday

Week 1 30 min 35 min 20 min 30 min 35 min

Week 2 20 min 40 min 20 min 35 min 30 min

Week 3 20 min 40 min 30 min 45 min 20 min

Week 4 30 min 45 min 20 min 30 min 45 min

This is flexible and will depend on how you are feeling and how your body is responding to the training. Any one of these days you could take as a rest day, continuing on the four-day routine or substitute running for some other activity.

I am a great believer in cross training, although some runners would disagree, so you could swim, cycle, do a gym workout, weights, yoga, or any other type of exercise you choose. Nothing is set in stone, but as this is about running, you do need to run at some stage to be a runner.

For those who want more, the next phase introduces hill work, speed play, and gives you the opportunity to take your running to the next level.

PHASE FIVE: Minimum of Four Weeks

Run on six days a week, as follows:

Monday: run 35–40 minutes, comfortable pace

Tuesday: run 30 minutes, including some hill work

Wednesday: run 35–40 minutes, including 10–15 minutes speed or tempo work! This could include undulation with 50 to 400-meter bursts.

Thursday: jog 30 minutes

Friday: rest

Saturday: run 30–45 minutes

Sunday: run 45–60 minutes

[12] STRETCHING FOR RUNNERS

Hamstrings

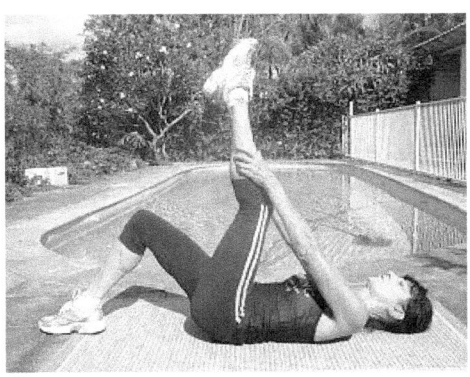

The hamstrings run from the buttocks to just below the knee, down the back of the leg. This muscle is responsible for lifting the lower leg and bending the knee after the quads have lifted the knee

1. Lay on your back, bending both legs looking up.

2. Keeping the small of the back pressed into the ground, lift the right leg up, clasping your

hands around the calf and straightening the leg up toward the ceiling until you feel the stretch in the hamstring.

3. Hold for 30 seconds and change legs.

If you are tight in the hamstring, do not try to force the stretch to the point of pain. This can cause injury. This goes for every muscle-stretching exercise.

Calf Gastrocnemius

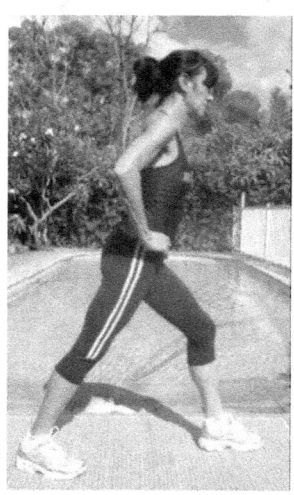

The gastrocnemius muscle is the larger of the two calf muscles.

1. Stand with your feet parallel to each other, toes pointing forward.

2. Take one leg forward, leaving the other behind, as if you are taking a step.

3. Lean forward, keeping the heel of the back foot on the ground, gently lean forward until you feel the stretch down the back of the calf.

4. Don't bounce or try to force the stretch.

5. Hold for 30 seconds, then change legs and repeat.

Calf Soleus

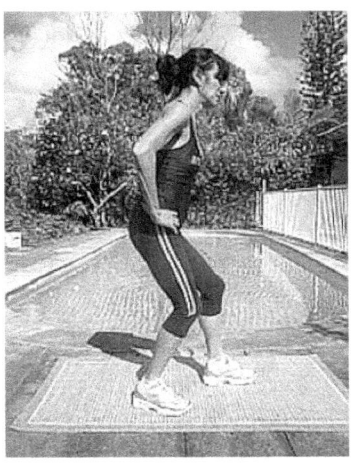

This is the other major calf muscle to stretch. This you need to sit down into the muscle.

1. Stand with both feet parallel and step back with the right leg, keeping the body upright and in alignment.

2. Make sure both feet are flat on the ground, facing forward.

3. Bend slightly at the knees as if you are going to sit on an imaginary chair, putting your weight into the back calf.

4. You should feel the stretch in your lower calf

5. Hold the stretch for 30 seconds, then change sides and repeat on the other leg.

Quadriceps

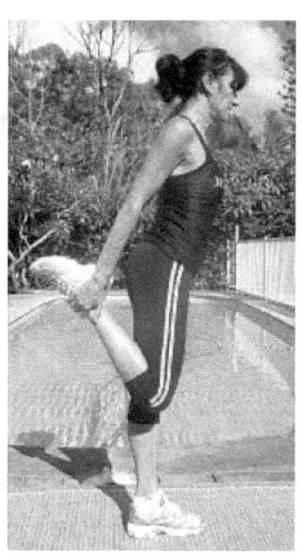

These are the muscles at the front of the thigh. They are responsible for straightening the leg.

1. Stand up straight, feet parallel and together.

2. Bend the right leg at the knee, reaching back with the right hand and grasping the ankle. You might wish to lean against something to keep your balance.

3. Your knees should remain together with the right knee pointing straight down.

4. Pull the right ankle into the buttock, feeling the stretch down the front of the thigh.

5. Hold the stretch for 30 seconds, then change legs.

Hip Flexors

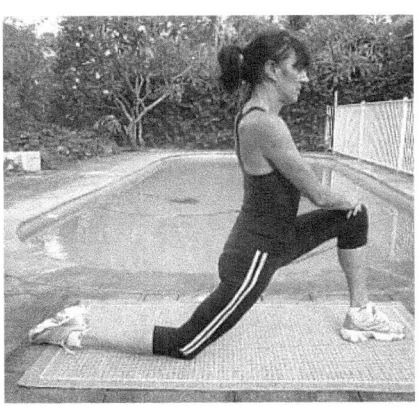

These muscles connect the lower spine and hip bone to the top of the thigh. Their main function is to lift the leg forward.

- 1. Take a long step forward with the right leg and let your left knee drop down toward the ground until it is on or just above the floor.

- 2. Your right knee should bend and be in alignment with your second toe

- 3. Keep your upper body straight and eyes look forward.

- 4. You should feel the stretch through the left hip.

- 5. Hold for 30 seconds, then change legs.

Iliotibial Band

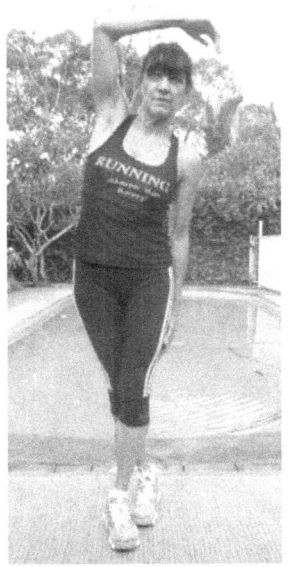

The iliotibial band runs from the hip down the side of the leg past the knee to the lower leg.

- 1. Cross your feet by putting one foot behind the other.

- 2. Keeping your body straight. lean in the same direction as the back leg. keeping the front knee slightly bent.

- 3. Take the arm on the side of the back leg and stretch it up above your head and over to the side.

- 4. Hold for 30 seconds, then change legs and repeat.

Groin

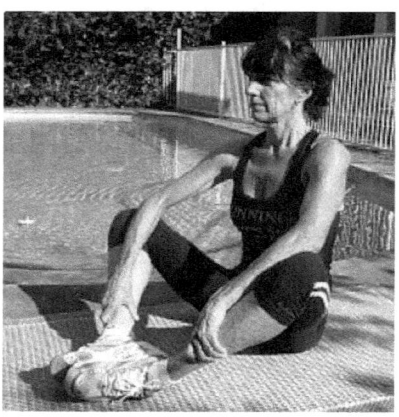

This stretches both sides of the groin.

1. Sitting, bend the knees and bring both feet in, putting the soles of the feet together.

2. Hold onto the ankles or feet with both hands and pull your lower back up and forward.

3. With your elbows, push out against the inside of your legs.

4. You should feel the stretch in the inner thighs.

5. Hold for 30 seconds.

If you are tight in this area, you might only manage to push your knees a short distance before you feel the pull, but as you do this regularly you will find you have a greater stretch.

Lower Back

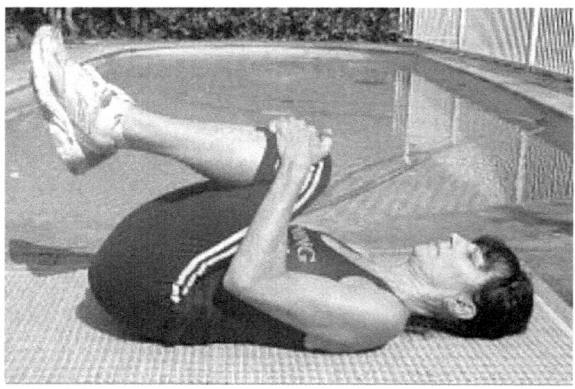

This stretches the lower part of the back.

1. Lie on your back, bringing both knees up to the chest.

2. Grasp the knees with both hands and pull them down toward the chest

3. You should feel the stretch in the lower back.

4. Hold for 30 seconds.

[13] CORE EXERCISES FOR RUNNERS

Side Plank

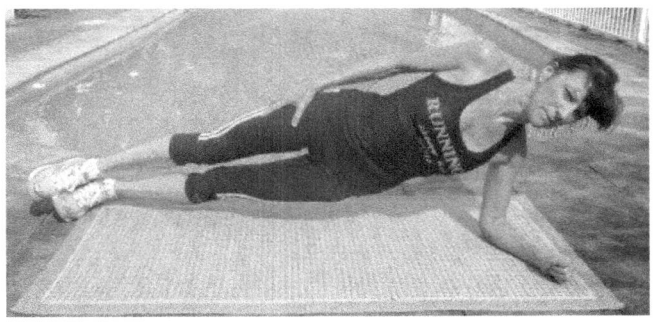

Works the obliques, transverse abdominals, back, hips, and glutes

1. Lay on your side and support your upper body with your forearm.

2. Lift your hips up off the ground, keeping your body weight supported, ensuring a

straight line from foot to shoulder. Don't let your hip drop down.

3. Extend your right arm straight up above your shoulder.

4. Hold this position for 20–30 seconds, then change sides

5. Repeat 10 times on each side.

Advanced: Support your body with your hand instead of your forearm

Plank Lift

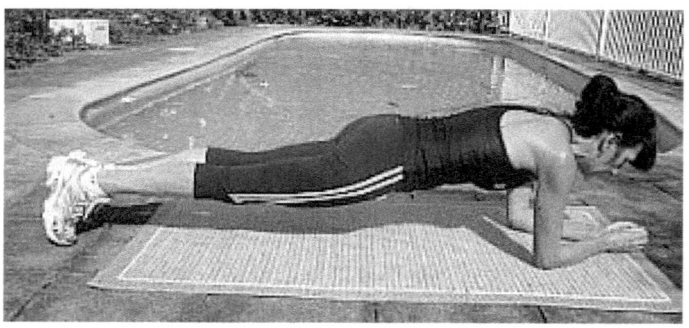

Works the transverse abdominals and back

1. Lay face down on the ground, prop yourself up onto your forearms with knees and feet together.

2. With your elbows beneath your shoulders, lift your torso, hips, and legs into a straight line off the ground, balancing on your toes and forearm.

3. Hold this position for 20–30 seconds.

Advanced: From this position lift one leg up off the ground, keeping the leg straight. Hold for 5 seconds, then lower. Do the same with the other leg. Repeat five to ten times.

Bridge

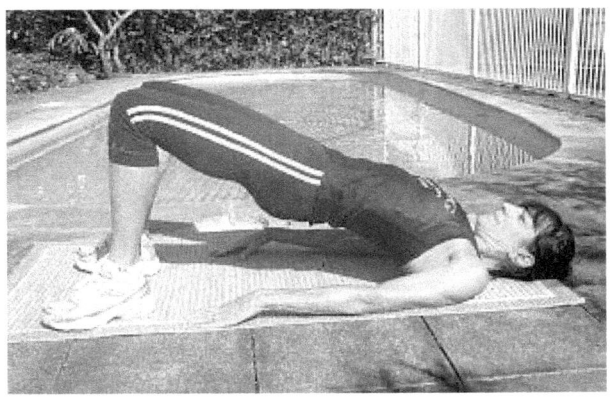

Works the glutes and hamstrings.

1. Lay on your back with knees bent to a 90-degree angle, feet flat on the ground.

2. Lift your butt off the ground until your body forms a straight line from your shoulders to your knees.

3. Hold for 5–10 seconds, then lower. Repeat ten times.

Advanced: Straighten one leg once hips are lifted.

Metronome

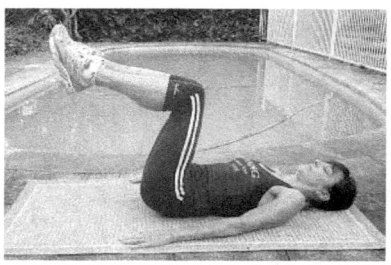

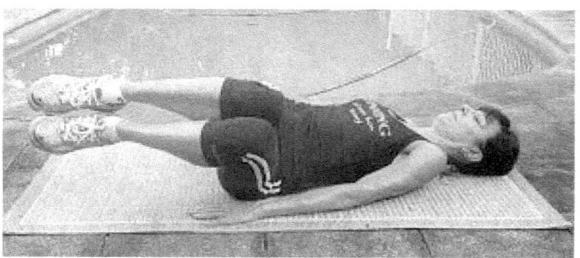

Works the obliques.

1. Lay on your back with knees bent and arms outstretched on the ground for support.

2. Raise your knees up over your hips with lower legs parallel to the ground, feet lifted.

3. Rotate your legs to the right, lowering your knees to as close to the floor as you can without lifting your left shoulder off the ground.

4. Return to the center and repeat on the left side, ensuring you are moving from your core and continue to move slowly from side to side.

5. Repeat ten times on each side.

Superman

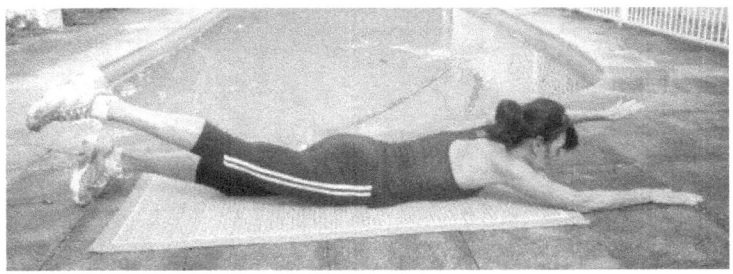

Works the transverse abdominals (deep abs) and lower back.

1. Lay face down on the ground with your arms and legs extended.

2. Raise your head, right arm, and left leg
    off the ground (as if you are flying,
    Superman style).

3. Hold for count of three, then lower.
    Repeat with the left arm and right leg.

4. Repeat tem times on each side.

Advanced: Lift both legs and arms together and hold
for the count of three. Lower and repeat ten times

[14] Dynamic Stretches

Leg Lift

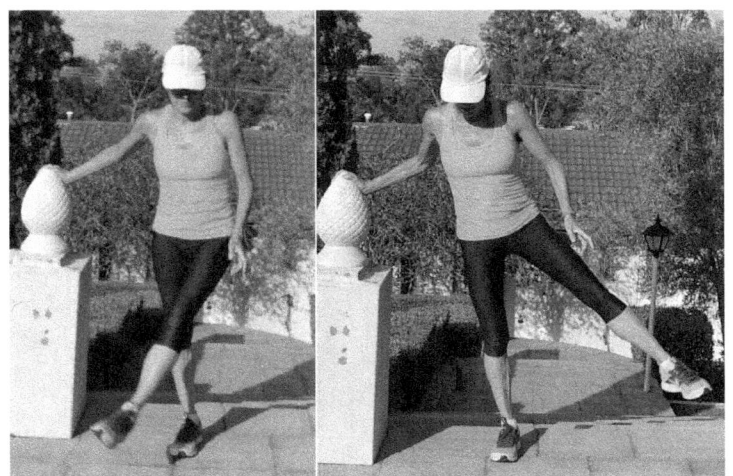

1. Swing one leg out to the side, then swing it back across the body in front of the other.

2. Repeat ten times on each side.

3. If you need something to balance, hold onto a steady object, such as a pole.

Butt Kick

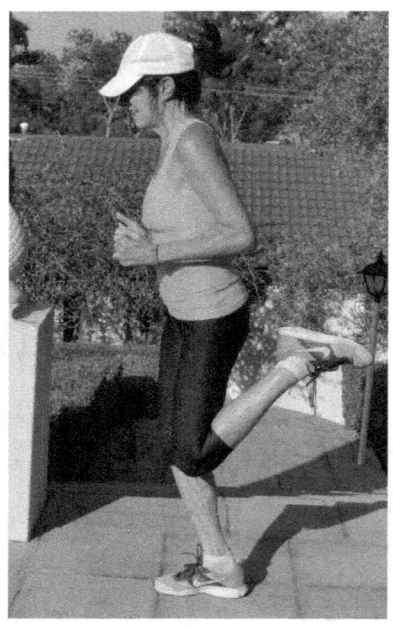

1. While standing tall, walk forward, swinging your back leg back and up to kick your butt.

2. Repeat with other leg.

Advanced: Do this butt-kicking exercise while jogging.

Toy Soldier

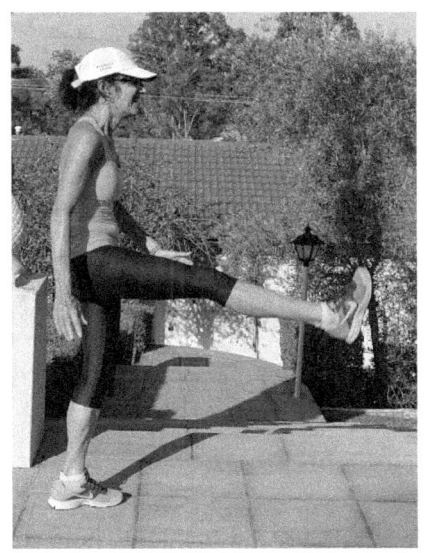

1. Keeping your back and knees straight, walk forward, lifting your leg straight out in front of you.

2. Flex your toes as you do this.

3. Repeat ten times on either side.

Advanced: Try doing it in a skipping motion.

Walking Lunges

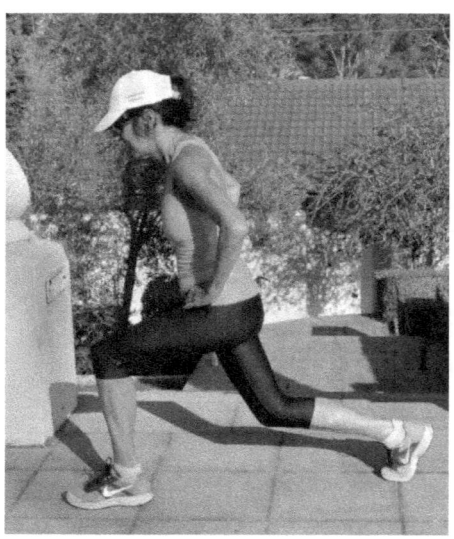

1. Step forward using a long stride, keeping the front knee just behind your toes.

2. Lower the body by dropping your back knee toward the ground.

3. Maintain an upright posture and keep your abdominal muscles tight.

4. Come back to standing position.

5. Repeat movement alternating sides ten times each.

Backward Lunges

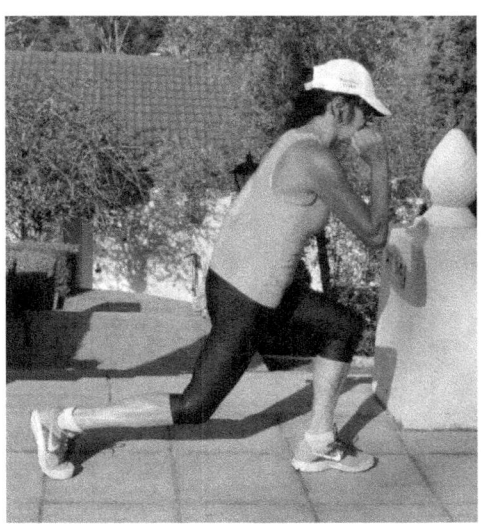

1. Step back, using a long stride, keeping the front knee just behind your toes.

2. Lower the body by dropping the back knee toward the ground.

3. Maintain an upright posture and keep abdominal muscles tight.

4. Come back to standing position.

5. Repeat movement alternating sides ten times each.

Leg Swings

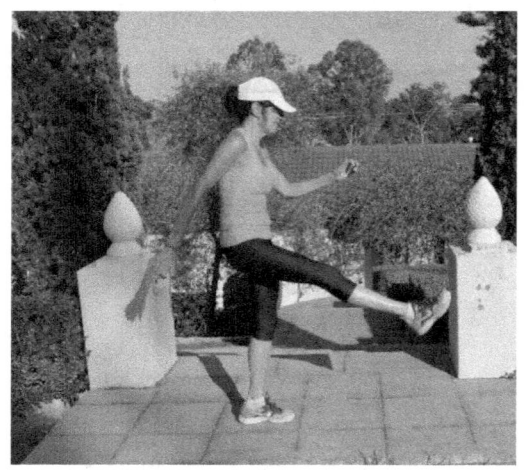

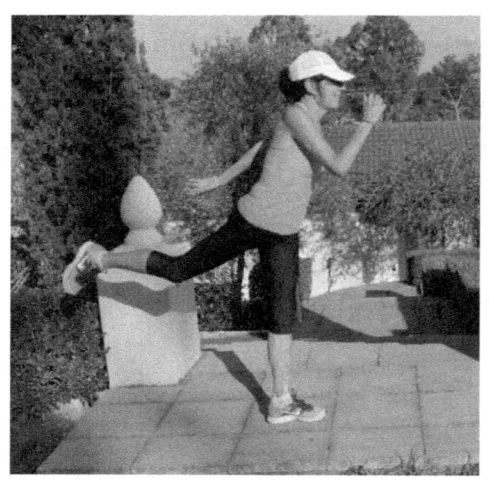

1. Standing on one leg, swing the other forward in front of you, then back behind you.

2. Hold onto something for support.

3. Repeat movement alternating sides ten times each.

High Knee Raises

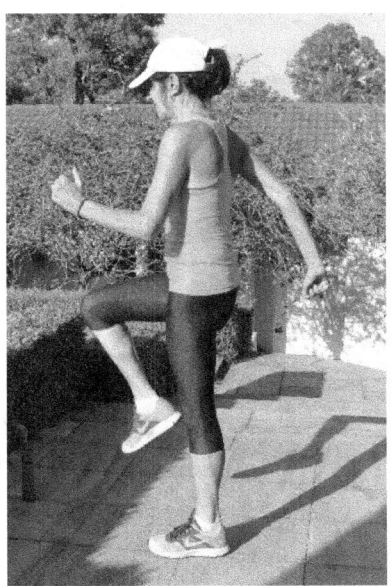

1. Stand with legs hip width apart

2. Lift your right knee towards your chest while your left remains firmly on the ground

3. Return your right foot back to the ground

4. Repeat with the left knee

5. Repeat movement alternating sides 10 times each

Advanced: Do above exercise but quickly as if running on the spot but with high knee lifts.

Side Lunges

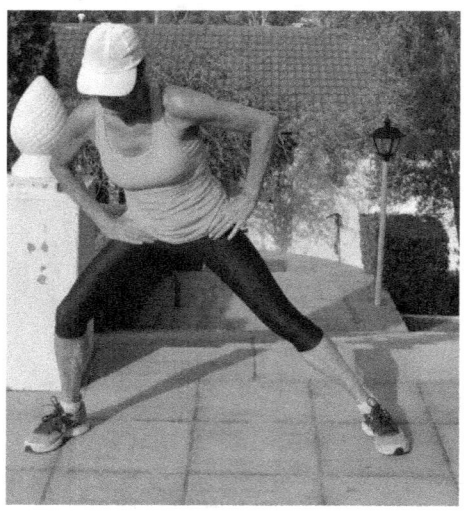

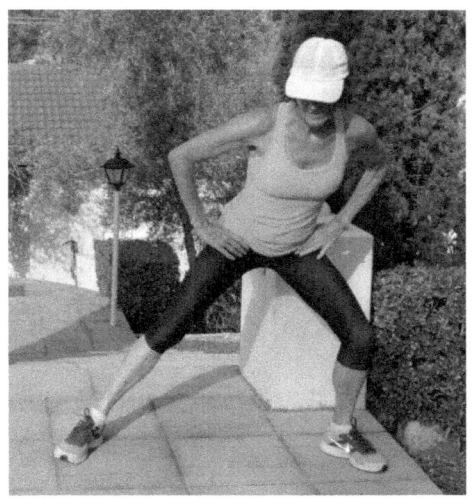

1. Standing with legs hip width apart
2. Take the right leg out to the side in a wide lunge
3. Return to standing position
4. Repeat with the left leg
5. Repeat movement alternating sides 10 times

Hip Rotation

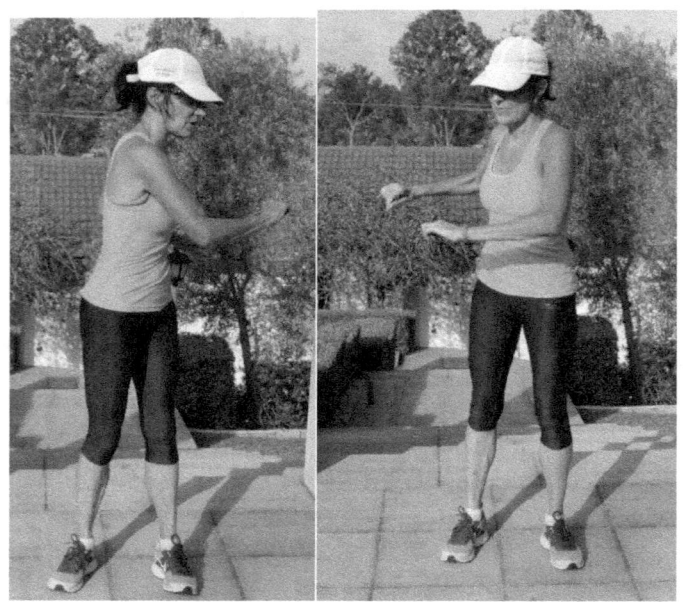

1. Standing straight with legs hip width apart
2. Rotate at the waist one way then the other
3. Repeat 10 times

This is just the beginning—
the rest is up to you!

ABOUT BERNICE FITZGIBBON

BERNICE FITZGIBBON is a health professional with a Diploma in Nursing, advanced qualification in Nursing specialising in sports science, health and wellness, as well as a qualified life coach, hypnotherapist and author.

She has over 35 years of experience in health and fitness, running competitively during her high school years and again at the seniors and masters level in road and cross-country athletics. She has run over 25 half marathons, one marathon and many off road trail runs.

Bernice has used her knowledge of health, exercise and running to encourage, motivate, and inform others to believe in themselves and not let perceived barriers and limited beliefs stop them from being the person they were always meant to be.

She has developed several web and social media sites to get her message across to others and to share her vast knowledge and experience in health, wellness and living a happy, healthy, and fulfilling life at any age.

RESOURCES

Websites

- About.com Sports Medicine
  www.sportsmedicine.about.com/

- Brendon Murray
  www.mezzanineca.com.au/

- Cool Running
  www.coolrunning.com/

- Hal Higdon's Marathon Training
  www.halhigdon.com/

- Irun the running hub
  http://www.irun.org.au/

- Medlineplus
  www.nlm.nih.gov/medlineplus/

- Peak Performance
  www.pponline.com.uk/

- <u>Runner's World</u>
  www.runnersworld.co.uk/
- Sporting Spirit Runners Manual
  www.sportingspirit.com.au/
- <u>Up and Running for Life</u>
  www.UpandRunningForLife.com/

Books

- *Running for Fitness* — Owen Barder
- *The Athlete's Book of Remedies* — Jordan D. Metzl, MD
- *The Complete Book of Running* — James Fixx
- *The Lydiard way RUN* — Arthur Lydiard

People

- Arthur Lydiard, coach of several New Zealand champions
- Bruce Milne, physiotherapist, athletics, New Zealand coach, and selector for New Zealand athletics
- Don Cameron, founder of the Christchurch Marathon Clinic, coach and mentor
- Pete Watts, club coach and mentor

YOUR THOUGHTS?

We love getting feedback from our readers and would really appreciate you taking a few minutes to post your comments or a brief review on our Amazon page.

Thank you!

.